Intuitive Eating

Journal

Improve your health, change
the relationship with food and
reconnect with your body.

Discover more tools and the motivation to change your life at:

https://en.angieramos.ca

Facebook: https://facebook.com/angie-Ramos-Life-Coaching-243163743246626/

Twitter: https://twitter.com/coachangieramos

Instagram: https://www.instagram.com/coachangieramos

Etsy: https://www.etsy.com/ca/shop/PositiveSpark

Cover designed by Starline / Freepik

Created by Angie Ramos, Life Coach
©Angie Ramos

ISBN: 9781794169418

Intuitive Eating Journal

A journal can help you to create a healthier and more positive lifestyle by changing unproductive habits and substituting them by empowering ones; it will help you to develop mindfulness by focusing on the positive stuff and improving your mindset by creating a gratitude practice.

Scientific evidence has shown that when you keep a journal, you get a positive impact on your mental and emotional well-being. Some of the benefits that you will experience are:

• Increase your self-esteem by knowing yourself better
• Clarify your ideas and feelings helping you to process and communicate complex ideas effectively
• Reduce stress when you write about your emotions and releasing all negativity about your day
• Increase your level of happiness by tracking your mood and identifying good patterns
• Improve your relationships as you look at things objectively

This Intuitive Eating Journal focuses on helping you to become more attuned to your body's natural hunger and fullness signals. You'll develop a better relationship with food and most importantly you will learn to trust your body and yourself.

If you have been struggling with dieting, emotional eating, or generally stressing about your weight and about food, this is a good start to change. It will help keep track of your feelings, to be more in tune with your hunger and fullness cues, and discover what foods keep you more satisfied and for how long.

I hope this journal helps you to finally forget about diets and to develop a new and better relationship with yourself.

I wish you success in all your endeavours,

Angie

I intend to accept my body today, love my body tomorrow, and appreciate my body always, no matter what my size is.

How to use your Intuitive Eating Journal

This Intuitive Eating Journal will help you build the foundations for a new relationship with food and with your body. Start feeling energized, nourished and happy about eating and around food.

Here are some ideas and strategies to follow so that you can start your Intuitive Eating Journey.

Identify foods that cause you stress or anxiety.
Choose 1-2 uncomfortable foods you identify each week to challenge the next one. Start with the one you feel the least anxious about and slowly work yourself up to the more challenging foods.

It is usually normal to eat more than you think is "acceptable" of any food you
choose to re-introduce. Give yourself permission to eat all the food and the quantity you want. The most important part of this is to not let any guilt or shame weigh you down.

Unconditional permission
Choose 2-3 times a week when you will choose to give yourself permission to eat and enjoy this food in a calm environment. Write down how you feel after eating, and repeat your positive intentions you listed on the commitment page.

Work on FULL PERMISSION to eat every single day for the rest of your life. It will take a while to sink in, but trust in the process and keep going.

Break the rules
In order to break the restrictive/overeating cycle you may be finding yourself in, it is so important to give up all food rules and create a positive mental space around food. Allow yourself to eat any food you would like without restriction or shame. With time this will allow you to tune into your own intuition and may make some of those foods less enticing with time.

Recognize the positive things about you and your body
Take this time to identify positive about yourself and about your body every day. To have some space throughout this journal to establish some positive intentions each morning as well as practice positive affirmations that could take you away from your negative self-talk. In doing this you will improve the relationship with your body and have a more positive mindset.

10 principles of Intuitive Eating

♡ REJECT THE DIET MENTALITY
Forget about diets that offer false hope of losing weight quickly. Reflect on how you felt when you were on a diet? Did you actually lose weight and kept it off? Does dieting feel good for you?

♡ HONOR YOUR HUNGER
Be mindful of your hunger and satiety cues. Nurture your body, keep it well fed with adequate energy and carbohydrates. If not you risk triggering your primal drive to overeat.

♡ MAKE PEACE WITH FOOD
Give yourself unconditional permission to eat. "I can't or I shouldn't eat this or that" leads to intense feelings of deprivation into cravings and, often, bingeing.

♡ CHALLENGE THE FOOD POLICE
Limit your negative self-talk and the rules you have about food. Your food choices don't determine your worthiness.

♡ RESPECT YOUR FULLNESS
Learn to identify when you are satisfied, listen to your body signals that tell you that you are no longer hungry. Avoid doing other activities while eating and pay attention to your body.

♡ DISCOVER THE SATISFACTION FACTOR
Enjoy your food, find pleasure in the experience of eating what you like. You will find that it takes much less food to decide you've had enough. The pleasure you'll find in the experience is crucial in helping you feel satisfied and content.

HONOR YOUR FEELINGS WITHOUT USING FOOD
Be aware of how you feel, develop emotional intelligence and find ways to comfort and nurture yourself. Try to resolve your issues without using food. Explore self-care and alternative ways to comfort yourself.

RESPECT YOUR BODY
Accept and love your body just as it is now. Stop being so critical about your body shape, learn to see the positive. Loving and respecting your body will help you to make choices about food and exercise that are logical, rather than emotional.

EXERCISE FEEL THE DIFFERENCE
Move your body in ways that bring you the most joy. Exercise because you love your body, not because you want to change it. Choose something you enjoy, like dancing, walking, running or yoga. Don't force yourself into doing something you don't enjoy.

HONOR YOUR HUNGER
Make food choices that honor your health and that make you feel well. You don't have to eat perfectly, you just have to create a new healthy and positive lifestyle. Choose foods that give you energy & make you feel great.

Awareness Checklist

This series of questions will help you develop awareness in the way you eat and how you feel while eating.

- ♡ Why am I eating?
- ♡ Am I really physically hungry? How do I feel?
- ♡ Am I eating because I was bored, stressed, or sad?
- ♡ Am I sitting while I eat?
- ♡ Am I eating fast or slow?
- ♡ Am I eating without paying attention or am I savouring each bite?
- ♡ Do I feel satisfied?
- ♡ What is my satiety level?
- ♡ Do I like what I'm eating?
- ♡ How do I feel when I'm eating?
- ♡ Am I doing another activity when I eat?
- ♡ How do I feel when I finished eating?
- ♡ Am I sleepy when I finish eating or do I feel energized?
- ♡ Did my mood change before, during or after eating? Did I feel better or worse?
- ♡ After eating did I feel happy, angry, depressed, anxious or bad?

Hunger and Fullness Discovery Scale

Before eating, check in with yourself to see where you are on the hunger scale. Ideally, it should be 3 or 4. After eating, check in again with yourself, work toward ending your meal at 6 or 7.

Do not let yourself get here. When you are very hungry it is difficult to regulate what you eat and it is easier to over-eat. At this point, you are too hungry to care what you eat.	**1**	Starving, dizzy, irritable
	2	Ravenous, unable to concentrate
It's time to eat.	**3**	Solid Hunger, Ready to eat
You have more self-control at this point. You can enjoy your food and listen to your body cues. Eating would be pleasurable at this moment.	**4**	Beginning signs of hunger
	5	Comfortable, neither hungy nor full
You feel content, comfortable, neither hungry nor full. This is the place where you need to acknowledge you are feeling satisfied.	**6**	Slightly Satisfied
	7	Satisfied
Respect your body and listen to it. Stop eating when is no longer enjoyable and you are already satisfied. You feel uncomfortable, clothes feel very tight, and you wish you hadn't eaten so much.	**8**	Full
	9	Very uncomfortably full
	10	Stuffed to the point of feeling sick

9

10 Reasons to create a healthy lifestyle

Motivation is a fundamental part to reach your health and weight goals. The most important part of this motivation is that it should be an internal motivation, in this case figuring out why you want to be healthy and/or lose weight. Take 15 minutes to find 10 reasons why is important to you to heal your relationship with food and your body.

Try to read these reasons continuously, ideally every day. This will help you to stay motivated and achieve what you really want.

Eat well,
Move daily,
Hydrate often,
Sleep lots,
Love your body

Repeat for LIFE

90-Days Wellness Goal Planner

	What is my goal? What do I want to live?	Why do I want to achieve this? How do I want to feel? How will my life change?
Health and physical self-care		
Emotional & spiritual self-care		
Intimate relationship		
Family & Friends		
Work & Career		
Finances & Economy		
Hobbies & Social Life		

90-Days Wellness Goal Planner

What do I need to change to accomplish it? What kind of mindset do I have to develop?	What tasks or activities do I need to do? What habits do I need to adopt?

Monthly Planning

From your 90-days goals choose 4 of them you are willing to achieve during this month.

Goal #1

....

....

Why am I committed to achieve it? What would I miss out on if I didn't achieve it?

....

....

What actions do I have to do to achieve it? What habits do I have to build to make it happen?

....

....

....

....

Goal #2

....

....

Why am I committed to achieve it? What would I miss out on if I didn't achieve it?

....

....

What actions do I have to do to achieve it? What habits do I have to build to make it happen?

....

....

....

Month: ....

Goal #1

....

....

Why am I committed to achieve it? What would I miss out on if I didn't achieve it?

....

....

What actions do I have to do to achieve it? What habits do I have to build to make it happen?

....

....

....

....

Goal #2

....

....

Why am I committed to achieve it? What would I miss out on if I didn't achieve it?

....

....

What actions do I have to do to achieve it? What habits do I have to build to make it happen?

....

....

....

....

Weekly Planning

What is my intention for this week?

	Monday	Tuesday	Wednesday	Thursday
Breakfast				
Lunch				
Dinner				
Snacks				
Workout				

Week: ....

What can I do to take care of myself?

....
....
....
....

Friday	Saturday	Sunday	Shopping list

Monday

Positive Affirmation

....

....

....

What is my intention for today?

....

....

....

Hours of sleep: .... How did I sleep?: ....

What did I eat / drink?

How did I feel before, during and after eating?

Breakfast

Hunger

Fullness

Lunch

Hunger

Fullness

Dinner

Hunger

Fullness

Snacks

Hunger

Fullness

Workout

Did I eat anything out of habit? Or did I eat something because I was feeling happy, stressed, bored or any other emotion?

....

....

....

Were there any events or situations that provoked food cravings? What cravings were they?

....

....

Did I try new foods today? Were there any foods I enjoyed eating?

....

....

What made me feel good today?

....

....

....

Positive habits

☐ ....
☐ ....
☐ ....
☐ ....
☐

Things I am grateful for

....

....

....

....

....

Tuesday

What do I love about my body?

....

....

....

Today is my opportunity to:

....

....

....

Hours of sleep: .... How did I sleep?: ....

	What did I eat / drink?		How did I feel before, during and after eating?
Breakfast		Hunger / Fullness	
Lunch		Hunger / Fullness	
Dinner		Hunger / Fullness	
Snacks		Hunger / Fullness	

Workout

Notice how many times throughout the day I talk negatively about myself. What are these thoughts?

....

....

....

....

What were some foods that caused me stress or anxiety? These foods may be the ones I most often avoid or feel guilt over after eating.

....

....

....

In what ways did I practice mindful eating today?

....

....

....

What made me feel good today?

....

....

....

....

Positive habits

☐ ....

☐ ....

☐ ....

☐ ....

☐ ....

Things I am grateful for

....

....

....

....

....

Wednesday

Motivational Quote

....

....

....

What does my ideal day look like?

....

....

....

Hours of sleep: .... How did I sleep?: ....

	What did I eat / drink?		How did I feel before, during and after eating?
Breakfast		Hunger ⬭ Fullness ⬭	
Lunch		Hunger ⬭ Fullness ⬭	
Dinner		Hunger ⬭ Fullness ⬭	
Snacks		Hunger ⬭ Fullness ⬭	

Workout

What food-rules I tended to repeat in my mind over and over. Where did these rules come from? Do they make me feel good or restricted?

....

....

....

What life would be like without these food rules? What would be different?

....

....

....

What did I notice about my mindset today?

....

....

What was the best thing that happened to me today?

....

....

....

Positive habits

☐ ....

☐ ....

☐ ....

☐ ....

☐ ....

Things I am grateful for

....

....

....

....

Thursday

Positive Affirmation

....

....

....

What are my unique gifts and talents?

....

....

....

Hours of sleep: .... How did I sleep?:

What did I eat / drink?

How did I feel before, during and after eating?

Breakfast

Hunger

Fullness

Lunch

Hunger

Fullness

Dinner

Hunger

Fullness

Snacks

Hunger

Fullness

Workout

Date: / / 20

What do I feel stressed, guilty or angry about? What do I do with these feelings?

What do I feel joyous, happy and abundant about? What do I do with these feelings?

What are 5 things that made me happy?

When do I feel the most in tune with myself?

Positive habits

☐
☐
☐
☐
☐

Things I am grateful for

Friday

Positive Affirmation

....

....

....

What is one positive thing you look forward today?

....

....

....

Hours of sleep: .... How did I sleep?: ....

	What did I eat / drink?		How did I feel before, during and after eating?
Breakfast		Hunger ⬭ Fullness ⬭	
Lunch		Hunger ⬭ Fullness ⬭	
Dinner		Hunger ⬭ Fullness ⬭	
Snacks		Hunger ⬭ Fullness ⬭	

Workout

What was my biggest challenge with food and body?

....

....

....

If I didn`t have these problems, how would my life be different?

....

....

....

How was my stress level lately? What can I do to support my body's stress response on a daily basis?

....

....

....

Dear body, I love you because ...

....

....

....

Positive habits

☐ ....
☐ ....
☐ ....
☐ ....
☐ ....

Things I am grateful for

....

....

....

....

....

Saturday

Positive Affirmation

....

....

....

When I look in the mirror, I feel...

....

....

....

Hours of sleep: .... How did I sleep?: ....

What did I eat / drink?

How did I feel before, during and after eating?

Breakfast

Hunger

Fullness

Lunch

Hunger

Fullness

Dinner

Hunger

Fullness

Snacks

Hunger

Fullness

Workout

What would life be like if I loved myself unconditionally? What would change?

....

....

....

....

What is one behaviour that is no longer serving me?

....

....

....

What are my strenghts?

....

....

What are my weaknesses?

....

....

....

Positive habits

☐ ....
☐ ....
☐ ....
☐ ....
☐ ....

Things I am grateful for

....

....

....

....

....

Sunday

Positive Affirmation

....

....

....

How could I relax today?

....

....

....

Hours of sleep: .... How did I sleep?:

What did I eat / drink?

How did I feel before, during and after eating?

Breakfast

Hunger

Fullness

Lunch

Hunger

Fullness

Dinner

Hunger

Fullness

Snacks

Hunger

Fullness

Workout

How do I feel when I eat mindfully, eating what I want, tasting & enjoying each bite until I'm satisfied?

....

....

....

....

Imagine what life would be like if you could love yourself unconditionally. What would that look like?

....

....

....

How could you create more space for self-love?

....

....

....

What gave a sense of satisfaction today?

....

....

....

....

Positive habits

☐ ....
☐ ....
☐ ....
☐ ....
☐ ....

Things I am grateful for

....

....

....

....

....

Weekly Review

On a scale from 1 to 10, how did I feel this week?

| 1 | 2 | 3 | 4 | 5 | 6 | 7 | 8 | 9 | 10 |

What were my 3 wins for the week?

....

....

....

....

What things I didn't like this week? What can I do to improve them?

....

....

....

....

What else can I do to improve my lifestyle?

....

....

....

....

How do I feel with my new lifestyle and my new mindset?

....

....

....

....

Weekly habit tracker

	Mon	Tue	Wed	Thu	Fri	Sat	Sun

Am I making progress? Am I embracing the change or resisting it?

....

....

....

Do I feel that my relationship with food is tied to stress and my emotions? What would my ideal relationship with food look like?

....

....

....

What are my current daily/weekly stressors? What can I do next week to reduce these stressors?

....

....

....

Weekly Planning

What is my intention for this week?

	Monday	Tuesday	Wednesday	Thursday
Breakfast				
Lunch				
Dinner				
Snacks				
Workout				

Week:

What can I do to take care of myself?

....

....

....

....

Friday	Saturday	Sunday	Shopping list

Monday

Positive Affirmation

....

....

....

What is my intention for today?

....

....

....

Hours of sleep: .... How did I sleep?: ....

	What did I eat / drink?		How did I feel before, during and after eating?

Breakfast

Hunger

Fullness

Lunch

Hunger

Fullness

Dinner

Hunger

Fullness

Snacks

Hunger

Fullness

Workout

36

Did I eat anything out of habit? Or did I eat something because I was feeling happy, stressed, bored or any other emotion?

....

....

....

....

Were there any events or situations that provoked food cravings? What cravings were they?

....

....

....

Did I try new foods today? Were there any foods I enjoyed eating?

....

....

....

What made me feel good today?

....

....

....

....

Positive habits

☐ ....

☐ ....

☐ ....

☐ ....

☐ ....

Things I am grateful for

....

....

....

....

....

Tuesday

What do I love about my body?

....

....

....

Today is my opportunity to:

....

....

....

Hours of sleep: .... How did I sleep?: ....

What did I eat / drink?   How did I feel before, during and after eating?

Breakfast

Hunger

Fullness

Lunch

Hunger

Fullness

Dinner

Hunger

Fullness

Snacks

Hunger

Fullness

Workout

Notice how many times throughout the day I talk negatively about myself. What are these thoughts?

....

....

....

....

What were some foods that caused me stress or anxiety? These foods may be the ones I most often avoid or feel guilt over after eating.

....

....

....

In what ways did I practice mindful eating today?

....

....

....

What made me feel good today?

....

....

....

....

Positive habits   Things I am grateful for

☐ ....

☐ ....

☐ ....

☐ ....

☐ ....

Wednesday

Motivational Quote

....
....
....

What does my ideal day look like?

....
....
....

Hours of sleep: .... How did I sleep?: ....

What did I eat / drink?		How did I feel before, during and after eating?

Breakfast

Hunger

Fullness

Lunch

Hunger

Fullness

Dinner

Hunger

Fullness

Snacks

Hunger

Fullness

Workout

What food-rules I tended to repeat in my mind over and over. Where did these rules come from? Do they make me feel good or restricted?

....

....

....

....

What life would be like without these food rules? What would be different?

....

....

....

....

What did I notice about my mindset today?

....

....

....

What was the best thing that happened to me today?

....

....

....

....

Positive habits

☐ ....

☐ ....

☐ ....

☐ ....

☐ ....

Things I am grateful for

....

....

....

....

....

Thursday

Positive Affirmation

....

....

....

What are my unique gifts and talents?

....

....

....

Hours of sleep: .... How did I sleep?:

What did I eat / drink?   How did I feel before, during and
                                                           after eating?

Breakfast

Hunger

Fullness

Lunch

Hunger

Fullness

Dinner

Hunger

Fullness

Snacks

Hunger

Fullness

Workout

What do I feel stressed, guilty or angry about? What do I do with these feelings?

....

....

....

What do I feel joyous, happy and abundant about? What do I do with these feelings?

....

....

....

What are 5 things that made me happy?

....

....

When do I feel the most in tune with myself?

....

....

....

Positive habits

☐ ....

☐ ....

☐ ....

☐ ....

☐ ....

Things I am grateful for

....

....

....

....

....

Friday

Positive Affirmation

....

....

....

What is one positive thing you look forward today?

....

....

....

Hours of sleep: .... How did I sleep?: ....

	What did I eat / drink?		How did I feel before, during and after eating?
Breakfast		Hunger / Fullness	
Lunch		Hunger / Fullness	
Dinner		Hunger / Fullness	
Snacks		Hunger / Fullness	

Workout

Date: / / 20

What was my biggest challenge with food and body?

....

....

....

If I didn`t have these problems, how would my life be different?

....

....

....

How was my stress level lately? What can I do to support my body's stress response on a daily basis?

....

....

Dear body, I love you because ...

....

....

....

Positive habits

- [ ] ....
- [ ] ....
- [ ] ....
- [ ] ....
- [ ]

Things I am grateful for

....

....

....

....

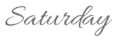

Saturday

Positive Affirmation

....

....

....

When I look in the mirror, I feel...

....

....

....

Hours of sleep: .... How did I sleep?: ....

What did I eat / drink?

How did I feel before, during and after eating?

Breakfast

Hunger

Fullness

Lunch

Hunger

Fullness

Dinner

Hunger

Fullness

Snacks

Hunger

Fullness

Workout

What would life be like if I loved myself unconditionally? What would change?

....

....

....

....

What is one behaviour that is no longer serving me?

....

....

....

....

What are my strenghts?

....

....

....

What are my weaknesses?

....

....

....

....

Positive habits	Things I am grateful for
☐	....
☐	....
☐	....
☐	....
☐	

Sunday

Positive Affirmation

How could I relax today?

Hours of sleep: How did I sleep?:

What did I eat / drink?

How did I feel before, during and after eating?

Breakfast

Hunger

Fullness

Lunch

Hunger

Fullness

Dinner

Hunger

Fullness

Snacks

Hunger

Fullness

Workout

How do I feel when I eat mindfully, eating what I want, tasting & enjoying each bite until I'm satisfied?

....

....

....

....

Imagine what life would be like if you could love yourself unconditionally. What would that look like?

....

....

....

How could you create more space for self-love?

....

....

....

What gave a sense of satisfaction today?

....

....

....

....

Positive habits

- ☐ ....
- ☐ ....
- ☐ ....
- ☐ ....
- ☐ ....

Things I am grateful for

....

....

....

....

....

Weekly Review

On a scale from 1 to 10, how did I feel this week?

| 1 | 2 | 3 | 4 | 5 | 6 | 7 | 8 | 9 | 10 |

What were my 3 wins for the week?

....

....

....

....

What things I didn't like this week? What can I do to improve them?

....

....

....

....

What else can I do to improve my lifestyle?

....

....

....

....

How do I feel with my new lifestyle and my new mindset?

....

....

....

....

Weekly habit tracker

	Mon	Tue	Wed	Thu	Fri	Sat	Sun

Am I making progress? Am I embracing the change or resisting it?

....

....

....

Do I feel that my relationship with food is tied to stress and my emotions? What would my ideal relationship with food look like?

....

....

....

What are my current daily/weekly stressors? What can I do next week to reduce these stressors?

....

....

....

Weekly Planning

What is my intention for this week?

....
....
....

	Monday	Tuesday	Wednesday	Thursday
Breakfast				
Lunch				
Dinner				
Snacks				
Workout				

Week: ....

What can I do to take care of myself?

....

....

....

....

Friday	*Saturday*	*Sunday*	*Shopping list*

Monday

Positive Affirmation

....
....
....

What is my intention for today?

....
....
....

Hours of sleep: .... How did I sleep?:

	What did I eat / drink?		How did I feel before, during and after eating?
Breakfast		Hunger / Fullness	
Lunch		Hunger / Fullness	
Dinner		Hunger / Fullness	
Snacks		Hunger / Fullness	

Workout

Did I eat anything out of habit? Or did I eat something because I was feeling happy, stressed, bored or any other emotion?

....

....

....

Were there any events or situations that provoked food cravings? What cravings were they?

....

....

Did I try new foods today? Were there any foods I enjoyed eating?

....

....

What made me feel good today?

....

....

....

Positive habits

- ☐ ....
- ☐ ....
- ☐ ....
- ☐ ....
- ☐

Things I am grateful for

....

....

....

....

....

Tuesday

What do I love about my body?

....

....

....

Today is my opportunity to:

....

....

....

Hours of sleep: ....   How did I sleep?: ....

What did I eat / drink?   How did I feel before, during and
                                             after eating?

Breakfast

Hunger

Fullness

Lunch

Hunger

Fullness

Dinner

Hunger

Fullness

Snacks

Hunger

Fullness

Workout

Notice how many times throughout the day I talk negatively about myself. What are these thoughts?

....

....

....

....

What were some foods that caused me stress or anxiety? These foods may be the ones I most often avoid or feel guilt over after eating.

....

....

....

In what ways did I practice mindful eating today?

....

....

....

What made me feel good today?

....

....

....

....

Positive habits	Things I am grateful for
☐	
☐	
☐	
☐	
☐	

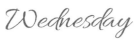

Wednesday

Motivational Quote

....

....

....

What does my ideal day look like?

....

....

....

Hours of sleep: .... How did I sleep?: ....

What did I eat / drink?   How did I feel before, during and
                                                          after eating?

Breakfast

Hunger

Fullness

Lunch

Hunger

Fullness

Dinner

Hunger

Fullness

Snacks

Hunger

Fullness

Workout

What food-rules I tended to repeat in my mind over and over. Where did these rules come from? Do they make me feel good or restricted?

....

....

....

What life would be like without these food rules? What would be different?

....

....

....

What did I notice about my mindset today?

....

....

What was the best thing that happened to me today?

....

....

....

Positive habits

☐ ....
☐ ....
☐ ....
☐ ....
☐ ....

Things I am grateful for

....

....

....

....

....

Thursday

Positive Affirmation

....

....

....

What are my unique gifts and talents?

....

....

....

Hours of sleep: .... How did I sleep?:

| | What did I eat / drink? | | How did I feel before, during and after eating? |

Breakfast

Hunger

Fullness

Lunch

Hunger

Fullness

Dinner

Hunger

Fullness

Snacks

Hunger

Fullness

Workout

What do I feel stressed, guilty or angry about? What do I do with these feelings?

....

....

....

....

What do I feel joyous, happy and abundant about? What do I do with these feelings?

....

....

....

....

What are 5 things that made me happy?

....

....

....

When do I feel the most in tune with myself?

....

....

....

....

Positive habits

☐ ....
☐ ....
☐ ....
☐ ....
☐ ....

Things I am grateful for

....

....

....

....

....

Friday

Positive Affirmation

....

....

....

What is one positive thing you look forward today?

....

....

....

Hours of sleep: .... How did I sleep?: ....

What did I eat / drink?

How did I feel before, during and after eating?

Breakfast

Hunger

Fullness

Lunch

Hunger

Fullness

Dinner

Hunger

Fullness

Snacks

Hunger

Fullness

Workout

What was my biggest challenge with food and body?

....
....
....

If I didn't have these problems, how would my life be different?

....
....
....

How was my stress level lately? What can I do to support my body's stress response on a daily basis?

....
....
....

Dear body, I love you because ...

....
....
....
....

Positive habits

☐ ....
☐ ....
☐ ....
☐ ....
☐ ....

Things I am grateful for

....
....
....
....
....

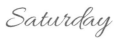

Saturday

Positive Affirmation

....

....

....

When I look in the mirror, I feel...

....

....

....

Hours of sleep: .... How did I sleep?: ....

	What did I eat / drink?		How did I feel before, during and after eating?
Breakfast		Hunger / Fullness	
Lunch		Hunger / Fullness	
Dinner		Hunger / Fullness	
Snacks		Hunger / Fullness	

Workout

What would life be like if I loved myself unconditionally? What would change?

....

....

....

....

What is one behaviour that is no longer serving me?

....

....

....

What are my strenghts?

....

....

....

What are my weaknesses?

....

....

....

....

Positive habits   Things I am grateful for

☐ ....

☐ ....

☐ ....

☐ ....

☐ ....

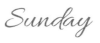

Sunday

Positive Affirmation

How could I relax today?

Hours of sleep: .... How did I sleep?: ....

What did I eat / drink?

How did I feel before, during and after eating?

Breakfast

Hunger

Fullness

Lunch

Hunger

Fullness

Dinner

Hunger

Fullness

Snacks

Hunger

Fullness

Workout

How do I feel when I eat mindfully, eating what I want, tasting & enjoying each bite until I'm satisfied?

Imagine what life would be like if you could love yourself unconditionally. What would that look like?

How could you create more space for self-love?

What gave a sense of satisfaction today?

Positive habits

- [ ]
- [ ]
- [ ]
- [ ]
- [ ]

Things I am grateful for

Weekly Review

On a scale from 1 to 10, how did I feel this week?

| 1 | 2 | 3 | 4 | 5 | 6 | 7 | 8 | 9 | 10 |

What were my 3 wins for the week?

What things I didn't like this week? What can I do to improve them?

What else can I do to improve my lifestyle?

How do I feel with my new lifestyle and my new mindset?

Weekly habit tracker

	Mon	Tue	Wed	Thu	Fri	Sat	Sun

Am I making progress? Am I embracing the change or resisting it?

....

....

....

Do I feel that my relationship with food is tied to stress and my emotions? What would my ideal relationship with food look like?

....

....

....

What are my current daily/weekly stressors? What can I do next week to reduce these stressors?

....

....

....

....

Weekly Planning

What is my intention for this week?

_____

_____

_____

	Monday	Tuesday	Wednesday	Thursday
Breakfast				
Lunch				
Dinner				
Snacks				
Workout				

Week:

What can I do to take care of myself?

....
....
....
....

Friday	Saturday	Sunday	Shopping list

Monday

Positive Affirmation

....
....
....

What is my intention for today?

....
....
....

Hours of sleep: .... How did I sleep?: ....

What did I eat / drink?

How did I feel before, during and after eating?

Breakfast

Hunger

Fullness

Lunch

Hunger

Fullness

Dinner

Hunger

Fullness

Snacks

Hunger

Fullness

Workout

72

Did I eat anything out of habit? Or did I eat something because I was feeling happy, stressed, bored or any other emotion?

....

....

....

....

Were there any events or situations that provoked food cravings? What cravings were they?

....

....

....

Did I try new foods today? Were there any foods I enjoyed eating?

....

....

....

What made me feel good today?

....

....

....

....

Positive habits   Things I am grateful for

☐ ....

☐ ....

☐ ....

☐ ....

☐ ....

Tuesday

What do I love about my body?

....

....

....

Today is my opportunity to:

....

....

....

Hours of sleep: .... How did I sleep?: ....

What did I eat / drink?

How did I feel before, during and after eating?

Breakfast

Hunger

Fullness

Lunch

Hunger

Fullness

Dinner

Hunger

Fullness

Snacks

Hunger

Fullness

Workout

74

Notice how many times throughout the day I talk negatively about myself. What are these thoughts?

....

....

....

....

What were some foods that caused me stress or anxiety? These foods may be the ones I most often avoid or feel guilt over after eating.

....

....

....

In what ways did I practice mindful eating today?

....

....

....

What made me feel good today?

....

....

....

....

Positive habits

- [ ] ....
- [ ] ....
- [ ] ....
- [ ] ....
- [ ] ....

Things I am grateful for

....

....

....

....

....

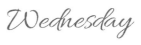
Wednesday

Motivational Quote

....

....

....

What does my ideal day look like?

....

....

....

Hours of sleep: .... How did I sleep?: ....

What did I eat / drink? How did I feel before, during and after eating?

Breakfast		Hunger / Fullness
Lunch		Hunger / Fullness
Dinner		Hunger / Fullness
Snacks		Hunger / Fullness

Workout

What food-rules I tended to repeat in my mind over and over. Where did these rules come from? Do they make me feel good or restricted?

....

....

....

....

What life would be like without these food rules? What would be different?

....

....

....

....

What did I notice about my mindset today?

....

....

....

What was the best thing that happened to me today?

....

....

....

....

Positive habits | Things I am grateful for

☐ .... | ....

☐ .... | ....

☐ .... | ....

☐ .... | ....

☐ .... |

Thursday

Positive Affirmation

....

....

What are my unique gifts and talents?

....

....

Hours of sleep: .... How did I sleep?: ....

	What did I eat / drink?		How did I feel before, during and after eating?
Breakfast		Hunger / Fullness	
Lunch		Hunger / Fullness	
Dinner		Hunger / Fullness	
Snacks		Hunger / Fullness	

Workout

What do I feel stressed, guilty or angry about? What do I do with these feelings?

....

....

....

What do I feel joyous, happy and abundant about? What do I do with these feelings?

....

....

....

What are 5 things that made me happy?

....

....

When do I feel the most in tune with myself?

....

....

....

Positive habits

☐ ....

☐ ....

☐ ....

☐ ....

☐ ....

Things I am grateful for

....

....

....

....

....

Friday

Positive Affirmation

....

....

....

What is one positive thing you look forward today?

....

....

....

Hours of sleep: .... How did I sleep?: ....

What did I eat / drink?   How did I feel before, during and after eating?

Breakfast

Hunger

Fullness

Lunch

Hunger

Fullness

Dinner

Hunger

Fullness

Snacks

Hunger

Fullness

Workout

What was my biggest challenge with food and body?

....

....

....

If I didn`t have these problems, how would my life be different?

....

....

....

How was my stress level lately? What can I do to support my body's stress response on a daily basis?

....

....

....

Dear body, I love you because ...

....

....

....

Positive habits	Things I am grateful for
☐	....
☐	....
☐	....
☐	....
☐	

Saturday

Positive Affirmation

....

....

When I look in the mirror, I feel...

....

....

....

Hours of sleep: .... How did I sleep?: ....

What did I eat / drink?

How did I feel before, during and after eating?

Breakfast

Hunger

Fullness

Lunch

Hunger

Fullness

Dinner

Hunger

Fullness

Snacks

Hunger

Fullness

Workout

What would life be like if I loved myself unconditionally? What would change?

....

....

....

....

What is one behaviour that is no longer serving me?

....

....

....

....

What are my strenghts?

....

....

....

What are my weaknesses?

....

....

....

....

Positive habits

☐ ....
☐ ....
☐ ....
☐ ....
☐ ....

Things I am grateful for

....

....

....

....

....

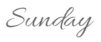

Sunday

Positive Affirmation

....

....

....

How could I relax today?

....

....

....

Hours of sleep: .... How did I sleep?: ....

	What did I eat / drink?		How did I feel before, during and after eating?
Breakfast		Hunger Fullness	
Lunch		Hunger Fullness	
Dinner		Hunger Fullness	
Snacks		Hunger Fullness	

Workout

How do I feel when I eat mindfully, eating what I want, tasting & enjoying each bite until I'm satisfied?

....

....

....

....

Imagine what life would be like if you could love yourself unconditionally. What would that look like?

....

....

....

How could you create more space for self-love?

....

....

....

What gave a sense of satisfaction today?

....

....

....

....

Positive habits

- [ ] ....
- [ ] ....
- [ ] ....
- [ ] ....
- [ ] ....

Things I am grateful for

....

....

....

....

....

Weekly Review

On a scale from 1 to 10, how did I feel this week?

| 1 | 2 | 3 | 4 | 5 | 6 | 7 | 8 | 9 | 10 |

What were my 3 wins for the week?

....

....

....

....

What things I didn't like this week? What can I do to improve them?

....

....

....

....

What else can I do to improve my lifestyle?

....

....

....

....

How do I feel with my new lifestyle and my new mindset?

....

....

....

....

Weekly habit tracker

	Mon	Tue	Wed	Thu	Fri	Sat	Sun

Am I making progress? Am I embracing the change or resisting it?

....

....

....

....

Do I feel that my relationship with food is tied to stress and my emotions? What would my ideal relationship with food look like?

....

....

....

What are my current daily/weekly stressors? What can I do next week to reduce these stressors?

....

....

....

....

Monthly Planning

From your 90-days goals choose 4 of them you are willing to achieve during this month.

Goal #1

....

....

Why am I committed to achieve it? What would I miss out on if I didn't achieve it?

....

....

What actions do I have to do to achieve it? What habits do I have to build to make it happen?

....

....

....

Goal #2

....

....

Why am I committed to achieve it? What would I miss out on if I didn't achieve it?

....

What actions do I have to do to achieve it? What habits do I have to build to make it happen?

....

....

....

Month: ....

Goal #1

....

....

Why am I committed to achieve it? What would I miss out on if I didn't achieve it?

....

....

What actions do I have to do to achieve it? What habits do I have to build to make it happen?

....

....

....

Goal #2

....

....

Why am I committed to achieve it? What would I miss out on if I didn't achieve it?

....

What actions do I have to do to achieve it? What habits do I have to build to make it happen?

....

....

....

....

Weekly Planning

What is my intention for this week?

	Monday	Tuesday	Wednesday	Thursday
Breakfast				
Lunch				
Dinner				
Snacks				
Workout				

Week: ....

What can I do to take care of myself?

....

....

....

....

Friday	*Saturday*	*Sunday*	*Shopping list*

Monday

Positive Affirmation

....

....

What is my intention for today?

....

....

Hours of sleep: ....   How did I sleep?: ....

	What did I eat / drink?		How did I feel before, during and after eating?
Breakfast		Hunger / Fullness	
Lunch		Hunger / Fullness	
Dinner		Hunger / Fullness	
Snacks		Hunger / Fullness	

Workout

Did I eat anything out of habit? Or did I eat something because I was feeling happy, stressed, bored or any other emotion?

....

....

....

....

Were there any events or situations that provoked food cravings? What cravings were they?

....

....

....

Did I try new foods today? Were there any foods I enjoyed eating?

....

....

....

What made me feel good today?

....

....

....

....

Positive habits	Things I am grateful for
☐	
☐	
☐	
☐	
☐	

Tuesday

What do I love about my body?

....

....

....

Today is my opportunity to:

....

....

....

Hours of sleep: .... How did I sleep?: ....

What did I eat / drink?

How did I feel before, during and after eating?

Breakfast

Hunger

Fullness

Lunch

Hunger

Fullness

Dinner

Hunger

Fullness

Snacks

Hunger

Fullness

Workout

94

Notice how many times throughout the day I talk negatively about myself. What are these thoughts?

....

....

....

....

What were some foods that caused me stress or anxiety? These foods may be the ones I most often avoid or feel guilt over after eating.

....

....

....

In what ways did I practice mindful eating today?

....

....

....

What made me feel good today?

....

....

....

....

Positive habits

☐ ....

☐ ....

☐ ....

☐ ....

☐ ....

Things I am grateful for

....

....

....

....

....

Wednesday

Motivational Quote

....

....

....

What does my ideal day look like?

....

....

....

Hours of sleep: .... How did I sleep?: ....

	What did I eat / drink?		How did I feel before, during and after eating?
Breakfast		Hunger ⬭ Fullness ⬭	
Lunch		Hunger ⬭ Fullness ⬭	
Dinner		Hunger ⬭ Fullness ⬭	
Snacks		Hunger ⬭ Fullness ⬭	

Workout

What food-rules I tended to repeat in my mind over and over. Where did these rules come from? Do they make me feel good or restricted?

....

....

....

....

What life would be like without these food rules? What would be different?

....

....

....

....

What did I notice about my mindset today?

....

....

....

What was the best thing that happened to me today?

....

....

....

....

Positive habits

Things I am grateful for

☐ ....

☐ ....

☐ ....

☐ ....

☐ ....

Thursday

Positive Affirmation

....

....

....

What are my unique gifts and talents?

....

....

....

Hours of sleep: ....   How did I sleep?:

What did I eat / drink?

How did I feel before, during and after eating?

Breakfast

Hunger

Fullness

Lunch

Hunger

Fullness

Dinner

Hunger

Fullness

Snacks

Hunger

Fullness

Workout

What do I feel stressed, guilty or angry about? What do I do with these feelings?

....

....

....

What do I feel joyous, happy and abundant about? What do I do with these feelings?

....

....

What are 5 things that made me happy?

....

....

When do I feel the most in tune with myself?

....

....

....

Positive habits	Things I am grateful for
☐	....
☐	....
☐	....
☐	....
☐	....

Friday

Positive Affirmation

....

....

....

What is one positive thing you look forward today?

....

....

....

Hours of sleep: .... How did I sleep?: ....

	What did I eat / drink?		How did I feel before, during and after eating?

Breakfast
Hunger
Fullness

Lunch
Hunger
Fullness

Dinner
Hunger
Fullness

Snacks
Hunger
Fullness

Workout

What was my biggest challenge with food and body?

....

....

....

If I didn`t have these problems, how would my life be different?

....

....

....

How was my stress level lately? What can I do to support my body's stress response on a daily basis?

....

....

Dear body, I love you because ...

....

....

....

....

Positive habits

☐ ....

☐ ....

☐ ....

☐ ....

☐ ....

Things I am grateful for

....

....

....

....

....

Saturday

Positive Affirmation

....

....

....

When I look in the mirror, I feel...

....

....

....

Hours of sleep: .... How did I sleep?: ....

What did I eat / drink?

How did I feel before, during and after eating?

Breakfast

Hunger

Fullness

Lunch

Hunger

Fullness

Dinner

Hunger

Fullness

Snacks

Hunger

Fullness

Workout

What would life be like if I loved myself unconditionally? What would change?

....

....

....

....

What is one behaviour that is no longer serving me?

....

....

....

....

What are my strenghts?

....

....

....

What are my weaknesses?

....

....

....

....

Positive habits

☐ ....
☐ ....
☐ ....
☐ ....
☐ ....

Things I am grateful for

....

....

....

....

....

Sunday

Positive Affirmation

....

....

How could I relax today?

....

....

....

Hours of sleep: .... How did I sleep?: ....

	What did I eat / drink?		How did I feel before, during and after eating?
Breakfast		Hunger / Fullness	
Lunch		Hunger / Fullness	
Dinner		Hunger / Fullness	
Snacks		Hunger / Fullness	

Workout

How do I feel when I eat mindfully, eating what I want, tasting & enjoying each bite until I'm satisfied?

....

....

....

Imagine what life would be like if you could love yourself unconditionally. What would that look like?

....

....

How could you create more space for self-love?

....

....

What gave a sense of satisfaction today?

....

....

....

Positive habits

☐ ....

☐ ....

☐ ....

☐ ....

☐ ....

Things I am grateful for

....

....

....

....

....

Weekly Review

On a scale from 1 to 10, how did I feel this week?

| 1 | 2 | 3 | 4 | 5 | 6 | 7 | 8 | 9 | 10 |

What were my 3 wins for the week?

....

....

....

....

What things I didn't like this week? What can I do to improve them?

....

....

....

....

What else can I do to improve my lifestyle?

....

....

....

....

How do I feel with my new lifestyle and my new mindset?

....

....

....

....

Weekly habit tracker

	Mon	Tue	Wed	Thu	Fri	Sat	Sun

Am I making progress? Am I embracing the change or resisting it?

....

....

....

....

Do I feel that my relationship with food is tied to stress and my emotions? What would my ideal relationship with food look like?

....

....

....

What are my current daily/weekly stressors? What can I do next week to reduce these stressors?

....

....

....

....

Weekly Planning

What is my intention for this week?

_____

_____

_____

_____

	Monday	Tuesday	Wednesday	Thursday
Breakfast				
Lunch				
Dinner				
Snacks				
Workout				

Week: ....

What can I do to take care of myself?

....
....
....
....

Friday	Saturday	Sunday	Shopping list

Monday

Positive Affirmation

....

....

....

What is my intention for today?

....

....

....

Hours of sleep: .... How did I sleep?: ....

What did I eat / drink?

How did I feel before, during and after eating?

Breakfast

Hunger

Fullness

Lunch

Hunger

Fullness

Dinner

Hunger

Fullness

Snacks

Hunger

Fullness

Workout

Did I eat anything out of habit? Or did I eat something because I was feeling happy, stressed, bored or any other emotion?

....

....

....

....

Were there any events or situations that provoked food cravings? What cravings were they?

....

....

....

Did I try new foods today? Were there any foods I enjoyed eating?

....

....

....

What made me feel good today?

....

....

....

....

Positive habits

☐ ....

☐ ....

☐ ....

☐ ....

☐ ....

Things I am grateful for

....

....

....

....

Tuesday

What do I love about my body?

....

....

....

Today is my opportunity to:

....

....

....

Hours of sleep: .... How did I sleep?: ....

What did I eat / drink?

How did I feel before, during and after eating?

Breakfast

Hunger

Fullness

Lunch

Hunger

Fullness

Dinner

Hunger

Fullness

Snacks

Hunger

Fullness

Workout

Notice how many times throughout the day I talk negatively about myself. What are these thoughts?

....

....

....

....

What were some foods that caused me stress or anxiety? These foods may be the ones I most often avoid or feel guilt over after eating.

....

....

....

In what ways did I practice mindful eating today?

....

....

....

What made me feel good today?

....

....

....

....

Positive habits

☐ ....
☐ ....
☐ ....
☐ ....
☐ ....

Things I am grateful for

....

....

....

....

....

Wednesday

Motivational Quote

....

....

....

What does my ideal day look like?

....

....

....

Hours of sleep: .... How did I sleep?: ....

	What did I eat / drink?		How did I feel before, during and after eating?

Breakfast

Hunger ⬭
Fullness ⬭

Lunch

Hunger ⬭
Fullness ⬭

Dinner

Hunger ⬭
Fullness ⬭

Snacks

Hunger ⬭
Fullness ⬭

Workout

What food-rules I tended to repeat in my mind over and over. Where did these rules come from? Do they make me feel good or restricted?

....

....

....

What life would be like without these food rules? What would be different?

....

....

....

What did I notice about my mindset today?

....

....

....

What was the best thing that happened to me today?

....

....

....

Positive habits

☐ ....
☐ ....
☐ ....
☐ ....
☐ ....

Things I am grateful for

....

....

....

....

....

Thursday

Positive Affirmation

....

....

....

What are my unique gifts and talents?

....

....

....

Hours of sleep: .... How did I sleep?: ....

	What did I eat / drink?		How did I feel before, during and after eating?
Breakfast		Hunger ◯ Fullness ◯	
Lunch		Hunger ◯ Fullness ◯	
Dinner		Hunger ◯ Fullness ◯	
Snacks		Hunger ◯ Fullness ◯	

Workout

What do I feel stressed, guilty or angry about? What do I do with these feelings?

....

....

....

What do I feel joyous, happy and abundant about? What do I do with these feelings?

....

....

....

What are 5 things that made me happy?

....

....

....

When do I feel the most in tune with myself?

....

....

....

....

Positive habits

☐ ....
☐ ....
☐ ....
☐ ....
☐ ....

Things I am grateful for

....

....

....

....

....

Friday

Positive Affirmation

....

....

....

What is one positive thing you look forward today?

....

....

....

Hours of sleep: .... How did I sleep?: ....

What did I eat / drink?		How did I feel before, during and after eating?

Breakfast

Hunger

Fullness

Lunch

Hunger

Fullness

Dinner

Hunger

Fullness

Snacks

Hunger

Fullness

Workout

What was my biggest challenge with food and body?

....

....

....

If I didn`t have these problems, how would my life be different?

....

....

....

How was my stress level lately? What can I do to support my body's stress response on a daily basis?

....

....

....

Dear body, I love you because ...

....

....

....

Positive habits

☐ ....
☐ ....
☐ ....
☐ ....
☐ ....

Things I am grateful for

....

....

....

....

....

Saturday

Positive Affirmation

....

....

....

When I look in the mirror, I feel...

....

....

....

Hours of sleep: .... How did I sleep?: ....

What did I eat / drink?

How did I feel before, during and after eating?

Breakfast

Hunger

Fullness

Lunch

Hunger

Fullness

Dinner

Hunger

Fullness

Snacks

Hunger

Fullness

Workout

What would life be like if I loved myself unconditionally? What would change?

....

....

....

....

What is one behaviour that is no longer serving me?

....

....

....

....

What are my strenghts?

....

....

....

What are my weaknesses?

....

....

....

....

Positive habits	Things I am grateful for
☐	....
☐	....
☐	....
☐	....
☐	....

Sunday

Positive Affirmation

....

....

How could I relax today?

....

....

Hours of sleep: .... How did I sleep?:

	What did I eat / drink?		How did I feel before, during and after eating?
Breakfast		Hunger ◯ Fullness ◯	
Lunch		Hunger ◯ Fullness ◯	
Dinner		Hunger ◯ Fullness ◯	
Snacks		Hunger ◯ Fullness ◯	

Workout

How do I feel when I eat mindfully, eating what I want, tasting & enjoying each bite until I'm satisfied?

....

....

....

....

Imagine what life would be like if you could love yourself unconditionally. What would that look like?

....

....

....

How could you create more space for self-love?

....

....

....

What gave a sense of satisfaction today?

....

....

....

....

Positive habits

☐ ....
☐ ....
☐ ....
☐ ....
☐ ....

Things I am grateful for

....

....

....

....

....

Weekly Review

On a scale from 1 to 10, how did I feel this week?

| 1 | 2 | 3 | 4 | 5 | 6 | 7 | 8 | 9 | 10 |

What were my 3 wins for the week?

....

....

....

....

What things I didn't like this week? What can I do to improve them?

....

....

....

....

What else can I do to improve my lifestyle?

....

....

....

....

How do I feel with my new lifestyle and my new mindset?

....

....

....

....

Weekly habit tracker

	Mon	Tue	Wed	Thu	Fri	Sat	Sun

Am I making progress? Am I embracing the change or resisting it?

....

....

....

....

Do I feel that my relationship with food is tied to stress and my emotions? What would my ideal relationship with food look like?

....

....

....

....

What are my current daily/weekly stressors? What can I do next week to reduce these stressors?

....

....

....

....

Weekly Planning

What is my intention for this week?

_____

_____

_____

_____

	Monday	Tuesday	Wednesday	Thursday
Breakfast				
Lunch				
Dinner				
Snacks				
Workout				

Week:

What can I do to take care of myself?

....
....
....
....

Friday	Saturday	Sunday	Shopping list

Monday

Positive Affirmation

....

....

What is my intention for today?

....

....

Hours of sleep: .... How did I sleep?: ....

What did I eat / drink?

How did I feel before, during and after eating?

	What did I eat / drink?	Hunger / Fullness	How did I feel before, during and after eating?
Breakfast		Hunger / Fullness	
Lunch		Hunger / Fullness	
Dinner		Hunger / Fullness	
Snacks		Hunger / Fullness	

Workout

Date: / / 20

Did I eat anything out of habit? Or did I eat something because I was feeling happy, stressed, bored or any other emotion?

....
....
....

Were there any events or situations that provoked food cravings? What cravings were they?

....
....

Did I try new foods today? Were there any foods I enjoyed eating?

....
....

What made me feel good today?

....
....
....

Positive habits

- ☐ ....
- ☐ ....
- ☐ ....
- ☐ ....
- ☐ ....

Things I am grateful for

....
....
....
....
....

Tuesday

What do I love about my body?

....

....

....

Today is my opportunity to:

....

....

....

Hours of sleep: .... How did I sleep?: ....

What did I eat / drink?

How did I feel before, during and after eating?

Breakfast

Hunger

Fullness

Lunch

Hunger

Fullness

Dinner

Hunger

Fullness

Snacks

Hunger

Fullness

Workout

Notice how many times throughout the day I talk negatively about myself. What are these thoughts?

....

....

....

....

What were some foods that caused me stress or anxiety? These foods may be the ones I most often avoid or feel guilt over after eating.

....

....

....

In what ways did I practice mindful eating today?

....

....

....

What made me feel good today?

....

....

....

....

Positive habits

☐ ....

☐ ....

☐ ....

☐ ....

☐ ....

Things I am grateful for

....

....

....

....

....

Wednesday

Motivational Quote

....

....

....

What does my ideal day look like?

....

....

....

Hours of sleep: .... How did I sleep?: ....

	What did I eat / drink?		How did I feel before, during and after eating?
Breakfast		Hunger / Fullness	
Lunch		Hunger / Fullness	
Dinner		Hunger / Fullness	
Snacks		Hunger / Fullness	

Workout

What food-rules I tended to repeat in my mind over and over. Where did these rules come from? Do they make me feel good or restricted?

....

....

....

....

What life would be like without these food rules? What would be different?

....

....

....

....

What did I notice about my mindset today?

....

....

....

What was the best thing that happened to me today?

....

....

....

....

Positive habits

- [ ] ....
- [ ] ....
- [ ] ....
- [ ] ....
- [ ] ....

Things I am grateful for

....

....

....

....

....

Thursday

Positive Affirmation

....

....

....

What are my unique gifts and talents?

....

....

....

Hours of sleep: .... How did I sleep?: ....

What did I eat / drink?

How did I feel before, during and after eating?

Breakfast

Hunger

Fullness

Lunch

Hunger

Fullness

Dinner

Hunger

Fullness

Snacks

Hunger

Fullness

Workout

What do I feel stressed, guilty or angry about? What do I do with these feelings?

....

....

....

What do I feel joyous, happy and abundant about? What do I do with these feelings?

....

....

....

What are 5 things that made me happy?

....

....

....

When do I feel the most in tune with myself?

....

....

....

....

Positive habits	Things I am grateful for
☐	....
☐	....
☐	....
☐	....
☐	....

Friday

Positive Affirmation

....

....

....

What is one positive thing you look forward today?

....

....

....

Hours of sleep: .... How did I sleep?: ....

	What did I eat / drink?		How did I feel before, during and after eating?
Breakfast		Hunger ⬭ Fullness ⬭	
Lunch		Hunger ⬭ Fullness ⬭	
Dinner		Hunger ⬭ Fullness ⬭	
Snacks		Hunger ⬭ Fullness ⬭	

Workout

What was my biggest challenge with food and body?

....

....

....

If I didn`t have these problems, how would my life be different?

....

....

....

How was my stress level lately? What can I do to support my body's stress response on a daily basis?

....

....

Dear body, I love you because ...

....

....

....

....

Positive habits

☐ ....
☐ ....
☐ ....
☐ ....
☐ ....

Things I am grateful for

....

....

....

....

Saturday

Positive Affirmation

....

....

....

When I look in the mirror, I feel...

....

....

....

Hours of sleep: .... How did I sleep?: ....

	What did I eat / drink?		How did I feel before, during and after eating?
Breakfast		Hunger ◯ Fullness ◯	
Lunch		Hunger ◯ Fullness ◯	
Dinner		Hunger ◯ Fullness ◯	
Snacks		Hunger ◯ Fullness ◯	

Workout

What would life be like if I loved myself unconditionally? What would change?

....

....

....

....

What is one behaviour that is no longer serving me?

....

....

....

What are my strenghts?

....

....

....

What are my weaknesses?

....

....

....

....

Positive habits

☐ ....
☐ ....
☐ ....
☐ ....
☐ ....

Things I am grateful for

....

....

....

....

....

Sunday

Positive Affirmation

....

....

....

How could I relax today?

....

....

....

Hours of sleep: .... How did I sleep?: ....

What did I eat / drink?

How did I feel before, during and after eating?

Breakfast

Hunger

Fullness

Lunch

Hunger

Fullness

Dinner

Hunger

Fullness

Snacks

Hunger

Fullness

Workout

How do I feel when I eat mindfully, eating what I want, tasting & enjoying each bite until I'm satisfied?

....

....

....

Imagine what life would be like if you could love yourself unconditionally. What would that look like?

....

....

How could you create more space for self-love?

....

....

What gave a sense of satisfaction today?

....

....

....

Positive habits

- ☐ ....
- ☐ ....
- ☐ ....
- ☐ ....
- ☐ ....

Things I am grateful for

....

....

....

....

....

Weekly Review

On a scale from 1 to 10, how did I feel this week?

| 1 | 2 | 3 | 4 | 5 | 6 | 7 | 8 | 9 | 10 |

What were my 3 wins for the week?

....

....

....

....

What things I didn't like this week? What can I do to improve them?

....

....

....

....

What else can I do to improve my lifestyle?

....

....

....

....

How do I feel with my new lifestyle and my new mindset?

....

....

....

....

Weekly habit tracker

	Mon	Tue	Wed	Thu	Fri	Sat	Sun

Am I making progress? Am I embracing the change or resisting it?

....

....

....

Do I feel that my relationship with food is tied to stress and my emotions? What would my ideal relationship with food look like?

....

....

....

What are my current daily/weekly stressors? What can I do next week to reduce these stressors?

....

....

....

....

Weekly Planning

What is my intention for this week?

....

....

....

....

	Monday	Tuesday	Wednesday	Thursday
Breakfast				
Lunch				
Dinner				
Snacks				
Workout				

Week: ....

What can I do to take care of myself?

....

....

....

....

Friday	Saturday	Sunday	Shopping list

Monday

Positive Affirmation

....

....

....

What is my intention for today?

....

....

....

Hours of sleep: .... How did I sleep?: ....

What did I eat / drink?

How did I feel before, during and after eating?

Breakfast

Hunger

Fullness

Lunch

Hunger

Fullness

Dinner

Hunger

Fullness

Snacks

Hunger

Fullness

Workout

Did I eat anything out of habit? Or did I eat something because I was feeling happy, stressed, bored or any other emotion?

....

....

....

....

Were there any events or situations that provoked food cravings? What cravings were they?

....

....

....

Did I try new foods today? Were there any foods I enjoyed eating?

....

....

....

What made me feel good today?

....

....

....

....

Positive habits

☐ ....

☐ ....

☐ ....

☐ ....

☐ ....

Things I am grateful for

....

....

....

....

....

Tuesday

What do I love about my body?

....

....

....

Today is my opportunity to:

....

....

....

Hours of sleep: .... How did I sleep?: ....

	What did I eat / drink?		How did I feel before, during and after eating?
Breakfast		Hunger ⬭ / Fullness ⬭	
Lunch		Hunger ⬭ / Fullness ⬭	
Dinner		Hunger ⬭ / Fullness ⬭	
Snacks		Hunger ⬭ / Fullness ⬭	

Workout

Notice how many times throughout the day I talk negatively about myself. What are these thoughts?

....

....

....

....

What were some foods that caused me stress or anxiety? These foods may be the ones I most often avoid or feel guilt over after eating.

....

....

....

In what ways did I practice mindful eating today?

....

....

....

What made me feel good today?

....

....

....

....

Positive habits

☐ ....
☐ ....
☐ ....
☐ ....
☐ ....

Things I am grateful for

....

....

....

....

....

Wednesday

Motivational Quote

....

....

....

What does my ideal day look like?

....

....

....

Hours of sleep: .... How did I sleep?: ....

What did I eat / drink?

How did I feel before, during and after eating?

Breakfast

Hunger

Fullness

Lunch

Hunger

Fullness

Dinner

Hunger

Fullness

Snacks

Hunger

Fullness

Workout

150

What food-rules I tended to repeat in my mind over and over. Where did these rules come from? Do they make me feel good or restricted?

....

....

....

What life would be like without these food rules? What would be different?

....

....

....

What did I notice about my mindset today?

....

....

What was the best thing that happened to me today?

....

....

....

Positive habits

☐ ....
☐ ....
☐ ....
☐ ....
☐ ....

Things I am grateful for

....

....

....

....

....

Thursday

Positive Affirmation

....

....

....

What are my unique gifts and talents?

....

....

....

Hours of sleep: .... How did I sleep?: ....

	What did I eat / drink?		How did I feel before, during and after eating?
Breakfast		Hunger ◯ Fullness ◯	
Lunch		Hunger ◯ Fullness ◯	
Dinner		Hunger ◯ Fullness ◯	
Snacks		Hunger ◯ Fullness ◯	

Workout

What do I feel stressed, guilty or angry about? What do I do with these feelings?

....

....

....

What do I feel joyous, happy and abundant about? What do I do with these feelings?

....

....

....

What are 5 things that made me happy?

....

....

....

When do I feel the most in tune with myself?

....

....

....

....

Positive habits   Things I am grateful for

☐ ....

☐ ....

☐ ....

☐ ....

☐ ....

Friday

Positive Affirmation

....

....

....

What is one positive thing you look forward today?

....

....

....

Hours of sleep: ....   How did I sleep?: ....

What did I eat / drink?

How did I feel before, during and after eating?

Breakfast

Hunger

Fullness

Lunch

Hunger

Fullness

Dinner

Hunger

Fullness

Snacks

Hunger

Fullness

Workout

What was my biggest challenge with food and body?

....

....

....

....

If I didn`t have these problems, how would my life be different?

....

....

....

....

How was my stress level lately? What can I do to support my body's stress response on a daily basis?

....

....

....

Dear body, I love you because ...

....

....

....

....

Positive habits

☐ ....

☐ ....

☐ ....

☐ ....

☐ ....

Things I am grateful for

....

....

....

....

....

Saturday

Positive Affirmation

....

....

When I look in the mirror, I feel...

....

....

Hours of sleep: .... How did I sleep?: ....

	What did I eat / drink?		How did I feel before, during and after eating?

Breakfast

Hunger ⬭
Fullness ⬭

Lunch

Hunger ⬭
Fullness ⬭

Dinner

Hunger ⬭
Fullness ⬭

Snacks

Hunger ⬭
Fullness ⬭

Workout

What would life be like if I loved myself unconditionally? What would change?

....

....

....

What is one behaviour that is no longer serving me?

....

....

....

What are my strenghts?

....

....

What are my weaknesses?

....

....

....

Positive habits	Things I am grateful for
☐	....
☐	....
☐	....
☐	....
☐	....

Sunday

Positive Affirmation

....

....

....

How could I relax today?

....

....

....

Hours of sleep: .... How did I sleep?: ....

What did I eat / drink?

How did I feel before, during and after eating?

Breakfast

Hunger

Fullness

Lunch

Hunger

Fullness

Dinner

Hunger

Fullness

Snacks

Hunger

Fullness

Workout

How do I feel when I eat mindfully, eating what I want, tasting & enjoying each bite until I'm satisfied?

....

....

....

....

Imagine what life would be like if you could love yourself unconditionally. What would that look like?

....

....

....

How could you create more space for self-love?

....

....

....

What gave a sense of satisfaction today?

....

....

....

....

Positive habits

☐ ....
☐ ....
☐ ....
☐ ....
☐ ....

Things I am grateful for

....

....

....

....

....

Weekly Review

On a scale from 1 to 10, how did I feel this week?

| 1 | 2 | 3 | 4 | 5 | 6 | 7 | 8 | 9 | 10 |

What were my 3 wins for the week?

....

....

....

....

What things I didn't like this week? What can I do to improve them?

....

....

....

....

What else can I do to improve my lifestyle?

....

....

....

....

How do I feel with my new lifestyle and my new mindset?

....

....

....

....

Weekly habit tracker

	Mon	Tue	Wed	Thu	Fri	Sat	Sun

Am I making progress? Am I embracing the change or resisting it?

....

....

....

Do I feel that my relationship with food is tied to stress and my emotions? What would my ideal relationship with food look like?

....

....

....

What are my current daily/weekly stressors? What can I do next week to reduce these stressors?

....

....

....

....

Monthly Planning

From your 90-days goals choose 4 of them you are willing to achieve during this month.

Goal #1

....

....

Why am I committed to achieve it? What would I miss out on if I didn't achieve it?

....

....

What actions do I have to do to achieve it? What habits do I have to build to make it happen?

....

....

....

Goal #2

....

....

Why am I committed to achieve it? What would I miss out on if I didn't achieve it?

....

....

What actions do I have to do to achieve it? What habits do I have to build to make it happen?

....

....

....

Month: ....

Goal #1

....

....

Why am I committed to achieve it? What would I miss out on if I didn't
achieve it?

....

....

What actions do I have to do to achieve it? What habits do I have to build
to make it happen?

....

....

....

Goal #2

....

....

Why am I committed to achieve it? What would I miss out on if I didn't
achieve it?

....

....

What actions do I have to do to achieve it? What habits do I have to build
to make it happen?

....

....

....

....

Weekly Planning

What is my intention for this week?

....

....

....

....

	Monday	Tuesday	Wednesday	Thursday
Breakfast				
Lunch				
Dinner				
Snacks				
Workout				

Week:

What can I do to take care of myself?

....

....

....

....

Friday	Saturday	Sunday	Shopping list

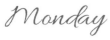
Monday

Positive Affirmation

....

....

....

What is my intention for today?

....

....

....

Hours of sleep: .... How did I sleep?: ....

What did I eat / drink?

How did I feel before, during and after eating?

Breakfast

Hunger

Fullness

Lunch

Hunger

Fullness

Dinner

Hunger

Fullness

Snacks

Hunger

Fullness

Workout

Did I eat anything out of habit? Or did I eat something because I was feeling happy, stressed, bored or any other emotion?

....

....

....

Were there any events or situations that provoked food cravings? What cravings were they?

....

....

....

Did I try new foods today? Were there any foods I enjoyed eating?

....

....

....

What made me feel good today?

....

....

....

....

Positive habits   Things I am grateful for

☐ ....

☐ ....

☐ ....

☐ ....

☐ ....

Tuesday

What do I love about my body?

....

....

....

Today is my opportunity to:

....

....

....

Hours of sleep: .... How did I sleep?: ....

	What did I eat / drink?		How did I feel before, during and after eating?
Breakfast		Hunger / Fullness	
Lunch		Hunger / Fullness	
Dinner		Hunger / Fullness	
Snacks		Hunger / Fullness	

Workout

Notice how many times throughout the day I talk negatively about myself. What are these thoughts?

....

....

....

What were some foods that caused me stress or anxiety? These foods may be the ones I most often avoid or feel guilt over after eating.

....

....

In what ways did I practice mindful eating today?

....

....

What made me feel good today?

....

....

....

Positive habits

- [ ] ....
- [ ] ....
- [ ] ....
- [ ] ....
- [ ]

Things I am grateful for

....

....

....

....

....

Wednesday

Motivational Quote

....

....

....

What does my ideal day look like?

....

....

....

Hours of sleep: .... How did I sleep?:

	What did I eat / drink?		How did I feel before, during and after eating?
Breakfast		Hunger ◯ Fullness ◯	
Lunch		Hunger ◯ Fullness ◯	
Dinner		Hunger ◯ Fullness ◯	
Snacks		Hunger ◯ Fullness ◯	

Workout

What food-rules I tended to repeat in my mind over and over. Where did these rules come from? Do they make me feel good or restricted?

....

....

....

What life would be like without these food rules? What would be different?

....

....

....

What did I notice about my mindset today?

....

....

....

What was the best thing that happened to me today?

....

....

....

Positive habits

- [ ] ....
- [ ] ....
- [ ] ....
- [ ] ....
- [ ] ....

Things I am grateful for

....

....

....

....

....

Thursday

Positive Affirmation

....

....

....

What are my unique gifts and talents?

....

....

....

Hours of sleep: .... How did I sleep?: ....

	What did I eat / drink?		How did I feel before, during and after eating?
Breakfast		Hunger ⬭ Fullness ⬭	
Lunch		Hunger ⬭ Fullness ⬭	
Dinner		Hunger ⬭ Fullness ⬭	
Snacks		Hunger ⬭ Fullness ⬭	

Workout

172

What do I feel stressed, guilty or angry about? What do I do with these feelings?

....

....

....

....

What do I feel joyous, happy and abundant about? What do I do with these feelings?

....

....

....

What are 5 things that made me happy?

....

....

....

When do I feel the most in tune with myself?

....

....

....

....

Positive habits

☐ ....

☐ ....

☐ ....

☐ ....

☐ ....

Things I am grateful for

....

....

....

....

....

Friday

Positive Affirmation

....

....

....

What is one positive thing you look forward today?

....

....

....

Hours of sleep: ....   How did I sleep?: ....

What did I eat / drink?   How did I feel before, during and after eating?

Breakfast

Hunger ⬭
Fullness ⬭

Lunch

Hunger ⬭
Fullness ⬭

Dinner

Hunger ⬭
Fullness ⬭

Snacks

Hunger ⬭
Fullness ⬭

Workout

What was my biggest challenge with food and body?

If I didn`t have these problems, how would my life be different?

How was my stress level lately? What can I do to support my body's stress response on a daily basis?

Dear body, I love you because ...

Positive habits

☐ ....
☐ ....
☐ ....
☐ ....
☐ ....

Things I am grateful for

Saturday

Positive Affirmation

....

....

....

When I look in the mirror, I feel...

....

....

....

Hours of sleep: .... How did I sleep?: ....

What did I eat / drink?

How did I feel before, during and after eating?

Breakfast

Hunger

Fullness

Lunch

Hunger

Fullness

Dinner

Hunger

Fullness

Snacks

Hunger

Fullness

Workout

What would life be like if I loved myself unconditionally? What would change?

....

....

....

....

What is one behaviour that is no longer serving me?

....

....

....

....

What are my strenghts?

....

....

....

What are my weaknesses?

....

....

....

....

Positive habits	Things I am grateful for
☐	....
☐	....
☐	....
☐	....
☐	

Sunday

Positive Affirmation

....
....

How could I relax today?

....
....

Hours of sleep: .... How did I sleep?: ....

	What did I eat / drink?		How did I feel before, during and after eating?
Breakfast		Hunger / Fullness	
Lunch		Hunger / Fullness	
Dinner		Hunger / Fullness	
Snacks		Hunger / Fullness	

Workout

How do I feel when I eat mindfully, eating what I want, tasting & enjoying each bite until I'm satisfied?

....

....

....

....

Imagine what life would be like if you could love yourself unconditionally. What would that look like?

....

....

....

How could you create more space for self-love?

....

....

....

What gave a sense of satisfaction today?

....

....

....

....

Positive habits

☐ ....
☐ ....
☐ ....
☐ ....
☐ ....

Things I am grateful for

....

....

....

....

....

Weekly Review

On a scale from 1 to 10, how did I feel this week?

| 1 | 2 | 3 | 4 | 5 | 6 | 7 | 8 | 9 | 10 |

What were my 3 wins for the week?

....

....

....

....

What things I didn't like this week? What can I do to improve them?

....

....

....

....

What else can I do to improve my lifestyle?

....

....

....

....

How do I feel with my new lifestyle and my new mindset?

....

....

....

....

Weekly habit tracker

	Mon	Tue	Wed	Thu	Fri	Sat	Sun

Am I making progress? Am I embracing the change or resisting it?

....

....

....

Do I feel that my relationship with food is tied to stress and my emotions? What would my ideal relationship with food look like?

....

....

....

What are my current daily/weekly stressors? What can I do next week to reduce these stressors?

....

....

....

Weekly Planning

What is my intention for this week?

....

....

....

....

	Monday	Tuesday	Wednesday	Thursday
Breakfast				
Lunch				
Dinner				
Snacks				
Workout				

Week:

What can I do to take care of myself?

Friday	Saturday	Sunday	*Shopping list*

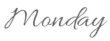

Monday

Positive Affirmation

....

....

....

What is my intention for today?

....

....

....

Hours of sleep: .... How did I sleep?: ....

What did I eat / drink?

How did I feel before, during and after eating?

Breakfast

Hunger

Fullness

Lunch

Hunger

Fullness

Dinner

Hunger

Fullness

Snacks

Hunger

Fullness

Workout

Did I eat anything out of habit? Or did I eat something because I was feeling happy, stressed, bored or any other emotion?

....

....

....

....

Were there any events or situations that provoked food cravings? What cravings were they?

....

....

....

Did I try new foods today? Were there any foods I enjoyed eating?

....

....

....

What made me feel good today?

....

....

....

....

Positive habits

☐ ....
☐ ....
☐ ....
☐ ....
☐ ....

Things I am grateful for

....
....
....
....
....

Tuesday

What do I love about my body?

....

....

Today is my opportunity to:

....

....

Hours of sleep: .... How did I sleep?: ....

What did I eat / drink?

How did I feel before, during and after eating?

Breakfast

Hunger

Fullness

Lunch

Hunger

Fullness

Dinner

Hunger

Fullness

Snacks

Hunger

Fullness

Workout

Notice how many times throughout the day I talk negatively about myself. What are these thoughts?

....

....

....

....

What were some foods that caused me stress or anxiety? These foods may be the ones I most often avoid or feel guilt over after eating.

....

....

....

In what ways did I practice mindful eating today?

....

....

....

What made me feel good today?

....

....

....

....

Positive habits

☐ ....
☐ ....
☐ ....
☐ ....
☐ ....

Things I am grateful for

....

....

....

....

....

Wednesday

Motivational Quote

....

....

....

What does my ideal day look like?

....

....

....

Hours of sleep: .... How did I sleep?: ....

	What did I eat / drink?		How did I feel before, during and after eating?
Breakfast		Hunger ⬭ Fullness ⬭	
Lunch		Hunger ⬭ Fullness ⬭	
Dinner		Hunger ⬭ Fullness ⬭	
Snacks		Hunger ⬭ Fullness ⬭	

Workout

What food-rules I tended to repeat in my mind over and over. Where did these rules come from? Do they make me feel good or restricted?

....

....

....

What life would be like without these food rules? What would be different?

....

....

....

What did I notice about my mindset today?

....

....

....

What was the best thing that happened to me today?

....

....

....

Positive habits

☐ ....
☐ ....
☐ ....
☐ ....
☐ ....

Things I am grateful for

....

....

....

....

....

Thursday

Positive Affirmation

....

....

....

What are my unique gifts and talents?

....

....

....

Hours of sleep: .... How did I sleep?: ....

What did I eat / drink?

How did I feel before, during and after eating?

Breakfast

Hunger

Fullness

Lunch

Hunger

Fullness

Dinner

Hunger

Fullness

Snacks

Hunger

Fullness

Workout

What do I feel stressed, guilty or angry about? What do I do with these feelings?

....

....

....

....

What do I feel joyous, happy and abundant about? What do I do with these feelings?

....

....

....

What are 5 things that made me happy?

....

....

....

When do I feel the most in tune with myself?

....

....

....

....

Positive habits

☐ ....

☐ ....

☐ ....

☐ ....

☐ ....

Things I am grateful for

....

....

....

....

....

Friday

Positive Affirmation

....

....

....

What is one positive thing you look forward today?

....

....

....

Hours of sleep: .... How did I sleep?: ....

What did I eat / drink?

How did I feel before, during and after eating?

Breakfast

Hunger

Fullness

Lunch

Hunger

Fullness

Dinner

Hunger

Fullness

Snacks

Hunger

Fullness

Workout

192

What was my biggest challenge with food and body?

....

....

....

If I didn't have these problems, how would my life be different?

....

....

....

How was my stress level lately? What can I do to support my body's stress response on a daily basis?

....

....

....

Dear body, I love you because ...

....

....

....

....

Positive habits	Things I am grateful for
☐	....
☐	....
☐	....
☐	....
☐	

Saturday

Positive Affirmation

....

....

....

When I look in the mirror, I feel...

....

....

....

Hours of sleep: .... How did I sleep?: ....

	What did I eat / drink?		How did I feel before, during and after eating?
Breakfast		Hunger ⬭ Fullness ⬭	
Lunch		Hunger ⬭ Fullness ⬭	
Dinner		Hunger ⬭ Fullness ⬭	
Snacks		Hunger ⬭ Fullness ⬭	

Workout

194

What would life be like if I loved myself unconditionally? What would change?

....

....

....

What is one behaviour that is no longer serving me?

....

....

....

What are my strenghts?

....

....

What are my weaknesses?

....

....

....

Positive habits

☐ ....
☐ ....
☐ ....
☐ ....
☐ ....

Things I am grateful for

....

....

....

....

....

Sunday

Positive Affirmation

....

....

How could I relax today?

....

....

Hours of sleep: .... How did I sleep?: ....

	What did I eat / drink?		How did I feel before, during and after eating?

Breakfast

Hunger

Fullness

Lunch

Hunger

Fullness

Dinner

Hunger

Fullness

Snacks

Hunger

Fullness

Workout

How do I feel when I eat mindfully, eating what I want, tasting & enjoying each bite until I'm satisfied?

....

....

....

Imagine what life would be like if you could love yourself unconditionally. What would that look like?

....

....

How could you create more space for self-love?

....

....

What gave a sense of satisfaction today?

....

....

....

Positive habits

☐ ....

☐ ....

☐ ....

☐ ....

☐ ....

Things I am grateful for

....

....

....

....

....

Weekly Review

On a scale from 1 to 10, how did I feel this week?

| 1 | 2 | 3 | 4 | 5 | 6 | 7 | 8 | 9 | 10 |

What were my 3 wins for the week?

....

....

....

....

What things I didn't like this week? What can I do to improve them?

....

....

....

What else can I do to improve my lifestyle?

....

....

....

How do I feel with my new lifestyle and my new mindset?

....

....

....

Weekly habit tracker

	Mon	Tue	Wed	Thu	Fri	Sat	Sun

Am I making progress? Am I embracing the change or resisting it?

....

....

....

....

Do I feel that my relationship with food is tied to stress and my emotions? What would my ideal relationship with food look like?

....

....

....

....

What are my current daily/weekly stressors? What can I do next week to reduce these stressors?

....

....

....

....

Weekly Planning

What is my intention for this week?

	Monday	Tuesday	Wednesday	Thursday
Breakfast				
Lunch				
Dinner				
Snacks				
Workout				

Week:

What can I do to take care of myself?

....

....

....

....

Friday	Saturday	Sunday	Shopping list

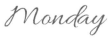

Monday

Positive Affirmation

....

....

....

What is my intention for today?

....

....

....

Hours of sleep: .... How did I sleep?: ....

What did I eat / drink?   How did I feel before, during and after eating?

Breakfast

Hunger

Fullness

Lunch

Hunger

Fullness

Dinner

Hunger

Fullness

Snacks

Hunger

Fullness

Workout

Did I eat anything out of habit? Or did I eat something because I was feeling happy, stressed, bored or any other emotion?

....

....

....

....

Were there any events or situations that provoked food cravings? What cravings were they?

....

....

....

Did I try new foods today? Were there any foods I enjoyed eating?

....

....

....

What made me feel good today?

....

....

....

....

Positive habits

☐ ....

☐ ....

☐ ....

☐ ....

☐ ....

Things I am grateful for

....

....

....

....

....

Tuesday

What do I love about my body?

....

....

....

Today is my opportunity to:

....

....

....

Hours of sleep: .... How did I sleep?: ....

What did I eat / drink?		How did I feel before, during and after eating?
Breakfast	Hunger / Fullness	
Lunch	Hunger / Fullness	
Dinner	Hunger / Fullness	
Snacks	Hunger / Fullness	

Workout

Notice how many times throughout the day I talk negatively about myself. What are these thoughts?

....

....

....

What were some foods that caused me stress or anxiety? These foods may be the ones I most often avoid or feel guilt over after eating.

....

....

In what ways did I practice mindful eating today?

....

....

What made me feel good today?

....

....

....

Positive habits

☐ ....
☐ ....
☐ ....
☐ ....
☐ ....

Things I am grateful for

....

....

....

....

....

Wednesday

Motivational Quote

....

....

....

What does my ideal day look like?

....

....

....

Hours of sleep: .... How did I sleep?: ....

	What did I eat / drink?		How did I feel before, during and after eating?
Breakfast		Hunger / Fullness	
Lunch		Hunger / Fullness	
Dinner		Hunger / Fullness	
Snacks		Hunger / Fullness	

Workout

What food-rules I tended to repeat in my mind over and over. Where did these rules come from? Do they make me feel good or restricted?

....

....

....

What life would be like without these food rules? What would be different?

....

....

....

What did I notice about my mindset today?

....

....

....

What was the best thing that happened to me today?

....

....

....

Positive habits

☐ ....

☐ ....

☐ ....

☐ ....

☐ ....

Things I am grateful for

....

....

....

....

Thursday

Positive Affirmation

....
....
....

What are my unique gifts and talents?

....
....
....

Hours of sleep: .... How did I sleep?: ....

	What did I eat / drink?		How did I feel before, during and after eating?
Breakfast		Hunger / Fullness	
Lunch		Hunger / Fullness	
Dinner		Hunger / Fullness	
Snacks		Hunger / Fullness	

Workout

What do I feel stressed, guilty or angry about? What do I do with these feelings?

....

....

....

....

What do I feel joyous, happy and abundant about? What do I do with these feelings?

....

....

....

What are 5 things that made me happy?

....

....

....

When do I feel the most in tune with myself?

....

....

....

....

Positive habits

☐ ....

☐ ....

☐ ....

☐ ....

☐ ....

Things I am grateful for

....

....

....

....

....

Friday

Positive Affirmation

....

....

....

What is one positive thing you look forward today?

....

....

....

Hours of sleep: .... How did I sleep?: ....

What did I eat / drink?

How did I feel before, during and after eating?

Breakfast
Hunger

Fullness

Lunch
Hunger

Fullness

Dinner
Hunger

Fullness

Snacks
Hunger

Fullness

Workout

210

What was my biggest challenge with food and body?

....

....

....

If I didn`t have these problems, how would my life be different?

....

....

....

How was my stress level lately? What can I do to support my body's stress response on a daily basis?

....

....

....

Dear body, I love you because ...

....

....

....

....

Positive habits

☐ ....

☐ ....

☐ ....

☐ ....

☐ ....

Things I am grateful for

....

....

....

....

Saturday

Positive Affirmation

....

....

....

When I look in the mirror, I feel...

....

....

....

Hours of sleep: .... How did I sleep?: ....

What did I eat / drink?

How did I feel before, during and after eating?

Breakfast

Hunger

Fullness

Lunch

Hunger

Fullness

Dinner

Hunger

Fullness

Snacks

Hunger

Fullness

Workout

What would life be like if I loved myself unconditionally? What would change?

....

....

....

What is one behaviour that is no longer serving me?

....

....

....

What are my strenghts?

....

....

....

What are my weaknesses?

....

....

....

Positive habits

☐ ....
☐ ....
☐ ....
☐ ....
☐ ....

Things I am grateful for

....

....

....

....

Sunday

Positive Affirmation

....

....

How could I relax today?

....

....

Hours of sleep: .... How did I sleep?: ....

What did I eat / drink?

How did I feel before, during and after eating?

Breakfast

Hunger

Fullness

Lunch

Hunger

Fullness

Dinner

Hunger

Fullness

Snacks

Hunger

Fullness

Workout

214

How do I feel when I eat mindfully, eating what I want, tasting & enjoying each bite until I'm satisfied?

....

....

....

....

Imagine what life would be like if you could love yourself unconditionally. What would that look like?

....

....

....

How could you create more space for self-love?

....

....

....

What gave a sense of satisfaction today?

....

....

....

....

Positive habits

☐ ....

☐ ....

☐ ....

☐ ....

☐ ....

Things I am grateful for

....

....

....

....

....

Weekly Review

On a scale from 1 to 10, how did I feel this week?

| 1 | 2 | 3 | 4 | 5 | 6 | 7 | 8 | 9 | 10 |

What were my 3 wins for the week?

....

....

....

....

What things I didn't like this week? What can I do to improve them?

....

....

....

....

What else can I do to improve my lifestyle?

....

....

....

....

How do I feel with my new lifestyle and my new mindset?

....

....

....

....

Weekly habit tracker

	Mon	Tue	Wed	Thu	Fri	Sat	Sun

Am I making progress? Am I embracing the change or resisting it?

....

....

....

....

Do I feel that my relationship with food is tied to stress and my emotions? What would my ideal relationship with food look like?

....

....

....

....

What are my current daily/weekly stressors? What can I do next week to reduce these stressors?

....

....

....

....

Weekly Planning

What is my intention for this week?

	Monday	Tuesday	Wednesday	Thursday
Breakfast				
Lunch				
Dinner				
Snacks				
Workout				

Week:

What can I do to take care of myself?

....

....

....

....

Friday	Saturday	Sunday	Shopping list

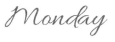

Monday

Positive Affirmation

....

....

....

What is my intention for today?

....

....

....

Hours of sleep: .... How did I sleep?: ....

What did I eat / drink? How did I feel before, during and after eating?

Breakfast

Hunger

Fullness

Lunch

Hunger

Fullness

Dinner

Hunger

Fullness

Snacks

Hunger

Fullness

Workout

Did I eat anything out of habit? Or did I eat something because I was feeling happy, stressed, bored or any other emotion?

....

....

....

....

Were there any events or situations that provoked food cravings? What cravings were they?

....

....

....

Did I try new foods today? Were there any foods I enjoyed eating?

....

....

....

What made me feel good today?

....

....

....

....

Positive habits

☐ ....

☐ ....

☐ ....

☐ ....

☐ ....

Things I am grateful for

....

....

....

....

....

Tuesday

What do I love about my body?

....

....

....

Today is my opportunity to:

....

....

....

Hours of sleep: .... How did I sleep?: ....

	What did I eat / drink?		How did I feel before, during and after eating?

Breakfast

Hunger

Fullness

Lunch

Hunger

Fullness

Dinner

Hunger

Fullness

Snacks

Hunger

Fullness

Workout

Notice how many times throughout the day I talk negatively about myself. What are these thoughts?

....

....

....

What were some foods that caused me stress or anxiety? These foods may be the ones I most often avoid or feel guilt over after eating.

....

....

In what ways did I practice mindful eating today?

....

....

What made me feel good today?

....

....

....

Positive habits

☐ ....
☐ ....
☐ ....
☐ ....
☐ ....

Things I am grateful for

....

....

....

....

....

Wednesday

Motivational Quote

....

....

....

What does my ideal day look like?

....

....

....

Hours of sleep: .... How did I sleep?: ....

What did I eat / drink?

How did I feel before, during and after eating?

Breakfast

Hunger

Fullness

Lunch

Hunger

Fullness

Dinner

Hunger

Fullness

Snacks

Hunger

Fullness

Workout

224

What food-rules I tended to repeat in my mind over and over. Where did these rules come from? Do they make me feel good or restricted?

....

....

....

....

What life would be like without these food rules? What would be different?

....

....

....

....

What did I notice about my mindset today?

....

....

....

What was the best thing that happened to me today?

....

....

....

....

Positive habits

☐ ....
☐ ....
☐ ....
☐ ....
☐ ....

Things I am grateful for

....

....

....

....

....

Thursday

Positive Affirmation

....

....

....

What are my unique gifts and talents?

....

....

Hours of sleep: ....   How did I sleep?: ....

What did I eat / drink?

How did I feel before, during and after eating?

Breakfast

Hunger

Fullness

Lunch

Hunger

Fullness

Dinner

Hunger

Fullness

Snacks

Hunger

Fullness

Workout

226

What do I feel stressed, guilty or angry about? What do I do with these feelings?

....

....

....

....

What do I feel joyous, happy and abundant about? What do I do with these feelings?

....

....

....

What are 5 things that made me happy?

....

....

When do I feel the most in tune with myself?

....

....

....

....

Positive habits

☐ ....
☐ ....
☐ ....
☐ ....
☐ ....

Things I am grateful for

....

....

....

....

....

Friday

Positive Affirmation

....

....

....

What is one positive thing you look forward today?

....

....

....

Hours of sleep: .... How did I sleep?: ....

	What did I eat / drink?		How did I feel before, during and after eating?

Breakfast

Hunger

Fullness

Lunch

Hunger

Fullness

Dinner

Hunger

Fullness

Snacks

Hunger

Fullness

Workout

What was my biggest challenge with food and body?

....

....

....

If I didn't have these problems, how would my life be different?

....

....

....

How was my stress level lately? What can I do to support my body's stress response on a daily basis?

....

....

Dear body, I love you because ...

....

....

....

Positive habits

☐ ....

☐ ....

☐ ....

☐ ....

☐ ....

Things I am grateful for

....

....

....

....

....

Saturday

Positive Affirmation

....

....

....

When I look in the mirror, I feel...

....

....

....

Hours of sleep: .... How did I sleep?: ....

What did I eat / drink?

How did I feel before, during and after eating?

Breakfast

Hunger

Fullness

Lunch

Hunger

Fullness

Dinner

Hunger

Fullness

Snacks

Hunger

Fullness

Workout

230

What would life be like if I loved myself unconditionally? What would change?

....

....

....

What is one behaviour that is no longer serving me?

....

....

....

What are my strenghts?

....

....

What are my weaknesses?

....

....

....

Positive habits

- ☐ ....
- ☐ ....
- ☐ ....
- ☐ ....
- ☐ ....

Things I am grateful for

....

....

....

....

....

Sunday

Positive Affirmation

....

....

How could I relax today?

....

....

....

Hours of sleep: .... How did I sleep?: ....

What did I eat / drink?   How did I feel before, during and after eating?

Breakfast

Hunger

Fullness

Lunch

Hunger

Fullness

Dinner

Hunger

Fullness

Snacks

Hunger

Fullness

Workout

How do I feel when I eat mindfully, eating what I want, tasting & enjoying each bite until I'm satisfied?

....

....

....

....

Imagine what life would be like if you could love yourself unconditionally. What would that look like?

....

....

....

How could you create more space for self-love?

....

....

....

What gave a sense of satisfaction today?

....

....

....

....

Positive habits	Things I am grateful for
☐	....
☐	....
☐	....
☐	....
☐	....

Weekly Review

On a scale from 1 to 10, how did I feel this week?

| 1 | 2 | 3 | 4 | 5 | 6 | 7 | 8 | 9 | 10 |

What were my 3 wins for the week?

....

....

....

....

What things I didn't like this week? What can I do to improve them?

....

....

....

....

What else can I do to improve my lifestyle?

....

....

....

....

How do I feel with my new lifestyle and my new mindset?

....

....

....

....

Weekly habit tracker

	Mon	Tue	Wed	Thu	Fri	Sat	Sun

Am I making progress? Am I embracing the change or resisting it?

....

....

....

Do I feel that my relationship with food is tied to stress and my emotions? What would my ideal relationship with food look like?

....

....

....

What are my current daily/weekly stressors? What can I do next week to reduce these stressors?

....

....

....

....

Notes

Notes

Notes

Notes

Notes

Notes

Notes

Notes

Notes